DILIGENTLY

DILIGENTLY

ARLINDA CHRISTINE

Dedication

To
Lisa Fuller and Nurse Brown
The Entire Staff At Christ Hospital
Aimee Tillet (With TriHealth)
Kim Youngblood
Don Mooney
Karen Imbus

There are not enough words to express my gratitude for your kindness, your thoughtfulness and your professionalism. Not only did each of you act in the manner in which you were trained, you also went above the call to ensure that I was safe, that I received assistance while in trauma and that I had safe spaces to heal. You all were part of my circle of safety in my time of trouble.

Namaste

God said: I'm restoring you as if it never happened.
(Instagram Post from @realtalkkim on November 10, 2019)

Preface

It's 1:45 a.m. on Saturday, August 3, 2019. Normally around this time of the year I am preparing for the upcoming school year, not this year. Right now, I'm working on uploading manuscripts, for my novel *Infused*, to be printed and reading through the final edited manuscript for this project, that I've affectionately entitled *Diligently*. The past nine months have been both difficult and yet encouraging. Just thinking that I will release *Diligently* nine months after I suffered a stroke is symbolic that God is about to birth something with this book, with my testimony and with my life.

DILIGENTLY

Today is May 21, 2019, and I am finally sitting down to organize my thoughts from over the past six months. After writing it in a journal, it was difficult to read it again. It felt as if I was reliving those emotions all over again, sending me to a sad place. So, I would just sit my notebook aside and wish for the courage to tell my story. The story of a woman who God allowed to be crushed in order to realize that her plans were not His plans, but now a time to live out her best life for His glory.

This time last year, I was helping students prepare for graduation and cleaning up my classroom to end the school year. If you would have told me last year that I'd be doing none of those things, I wouldn't have believed you.

Yet here I am; resigned from a career that I loved and recovering from a stroke. Yes; a stroke. Sometimes I have to say the word over and over again to fully understand it. My journey in the last six months has been stressful, hurtful, heartbreaking and at times, depressing. Nevertheless, through it all, my faith stayed fixed on God's love for me.

My prayer is that my experience blesses someone growing through similar experiences and that they will see a glimpse of hope to endure adversities and to later be a light for someone else.

But without faith it is impossible to please him: for he that cometh to God must believe that he is, and that he is a rewarder of them that diligently seek him.

Hebrews 11:6 (AKJV)

Halloween 2018

Lying across the bed on Halloween evening, I was doing one of my favorite pastimes that I love: talking to my mom on the phone. But, something prompted me to check my email account from work. As soon as I opened it, I saw the word, "Reassigned." I pressed the link for the email, read it to myself and then aloud to my mom. Immediately, she could hear that I was upset. I told her I had to get off the phone and when I did, I cried and cried. My youngest son, who had recently turned 13, was sitting near me and held me as I wept. I had been in my current position for 10 years and this year was to be my 17th year with the district.

Not only were my students very important to me, but I had grown to love serving overaged and credit deficient students with disabilities. Over the years, assisting underserved students with graduating from high school and finding employment became my passion. Moreover, this passion was ignited after learning more about The School To Prison Pipeline, after watching a video by The Children's Defense Fund, and the over identification of male students of color in special education. My students had not performed well in a traditional educational setting. Coming to our program gave them another chance and a different route to obtain their high school diploma and gainful employment.

Now, because our enrollment was low, I was being sent elsewhere. As I sat on my bed crying, I thought about my students, "How was I going to tell them?" For many of them, I was their confidant, to discuss life crisis with or to simply say hello and tell me about their weekend. My next thought was, "How do I shut down a classroom where I had been a teacher for ten years?" I was given two days to shut down and pack up my room, get students' grades together, and help my students process that I was leaving. In that moment, I couldn't figure out how to help them process something that I didn't even understand.

Once the tears stopped falling, I texted my paraprofessional. I've always jokingly called him the real teacher in our room. He's so amazing in the classroom and I know that he is going to be an incredible teacher. I shared all that I knew of my reassignment, and told him that I needed his organization and expertise to help me with my two-day moving endeavor. I made a few more phone calls and afterwards sat on my bed and focused on the tasks at hand. I knew it was going to be a rough process. Though looking back, I had no idea how hard it would actually be. All I had was my faith in knowing *that all things work together for good to them that love God, to them who are the called according to his purpose* (Romans 8:28 KJV).

November 1, 2018

In my mind, I had come up with a foolproof plan to take down all of my Pinterest-inspired decorations. After being moved from our former location to make room for a new school for gifted students, to a location that was dull and uninviting to students, I committed to creating a bright space where students would learn in a colorful and welcoming environment. Not only did I teach English, American Government and Economics to my students, I also introduced them to mindfulness and meditation. Mr. Bailey, my para, and I worked hard to create an inviting place for our students.

After I had taken all of the decorations down, a student walked into my room and asked me what I was doing. I felt a breath of both frustration and regret. Now, I should have contacted his family. This student had been through so much already. Our bond was unique in that he would just pop into my classroom for no reason at all. It didn't take long to sense that he found a connection to me as a mom, since he had lost his several years ago. If he were my son, he would've been my middle child because he fit perfectly between my two sons.

I stopped as I balled up the colorful tissue paper and gently told him that I was leaving. He laughed and asked me to stop playing. He stood in my classroom and stared at me and said, "You're lying." In the calmest voice that I could muster up, I told him about the program's numbers being low and that I was being reassigned to another school. Before I could get my thoughts completely out, he abruptly left my room in tears.

"Dag!" I thought. "This is going to be so hard."

At 8:20 a.m., the first bell rang and students entered my room. I taught English for the first three bells, but my first bell contained students that I had had the longest. It was really important that they learned of my leaving from me. The plan was to tell them that I was leaving and let them know that their new schedule would begin that very same day. I made another announcement that morning to stoic faces. I informed them that I wouldn't be having class that morning, since I needed to pack up my room. Next, I told them to follow their new schedule.

It felt like my students took on a Colin Kaepernick moment as they all got up, went and grabbed their unfinished work from the previous day. I looked over at Mr. Bailey and he put up "Webster's Word of the Day" on the screen and began playing mindful music through the classroom speakers.

I totally understood how they were feeling. They were hurt and had no intention of leaving my classroom. I went to my desk and cried, just like I am right now as I relive that moment. Later as I recovered, I would learn why leaving hurt so bad. The success of my students meant as much to me as the success of my own children.

November 2, 2018

The day before, I went home mentally drained. Fortunately, Enjoli came over to install a new hairstyle. Besides, sitting and talking with her would settle me down from such a rough week. I had rocked my natural look for about a month out of a challenge to myself. I actually loved it, but I figured I needed to switch things up as I prepared for my new adventure.

On my last day at the STEP Program, I allowed my students to come and go throughout the morning as normal. When they asked me who would teach them about mindfulness and play mindful music, I jokingly told them that they had to leave. Truthfully, I really needed them to leave my room, primarily because I didn't want them to see me sad. It was so hard to pack, console them and keep searching for tissues for all of us.

By the end of fourth bell, I was finished shutting my room down. I planned to have lunch with my students, just to sit and talk to them one last time. The more I planned, the harder it was to face them. After lunch, they all went to another classroom. But the moment had arrived. I walked into the classroom and tried to talk to them, and again I broke down and returned to my classroom. I went back to my room so incredibly hurt.

I kept looking at the clock; the hands seemed to be moving faster that day. With 15 minutes left in the day, I asked the students to come to my classroom. I needed a moment alone with just them. I really wanted them to hear my heart and encourage them to stay the course. We gathered in a small circle and I told them how proud I was of each of them. There were several new faces to the program, yet you would have thought I'd been their teacher for years.

I allowed them to speak from their hearts and told them it was okay to cry when you're hurting. I assured them that everything would be alright. That moment will stay in my heart forever. As my last task as their teacher, I walked them to the door one final time. Once all of the goodbyes and silly jokes were finished, I went to say goodbye to my fellow coworkers.

Earlier in the day, Mr. Bailey, along with some students, had packed my car. Now my car was filled with ten years of my teaching career and a huge part of my heart. I didn't know what was to come next. I just knew that my time at STEP was over.

That Weekend

I don't remember much about that weekend except that I slept a lot. Just going through the motions is what I can best describe that weekend. There was so much I wanted to know. What grades would I be working with? Would it be inclusion or small groups? I knew nothing about the school I had been reassigned to, nor had anyone contacted me from the school to tell me what my assignment was.

In my mind, I came up with a list of positive aspects concerning this move. It was a school with a late start and my youngest son had started basketball season. With me working at a school that dismissed later, I had time to shop at the Oakley Kroger. I also could stop periodically at Yagoot, Tyler's favorite yogurt, and surprise him with a 20-ounce smoothie with sliced bananas and strawberries.

Tyler's school was in the Eastern Conference and most of their games were closer to my newly assigned school. On game days, I could hop in my car and drive up 71 North or take Red Bank Road to games that were closer.

"Hmmmmm," I thought. "Just maybe this assignment is a blessing in disguise."

Then, Monday came.

November 5, 2018

On Monday, November 5th, I woke with a "Well, here we go!" attitude. I didn't sleep well that night at all—awakening several times throughout the night. After dropping Tyler off at school, I had over an hour until my new school started. I decided to make a couple of stops to kill the time.

I drove to the Kroger gas station on Montgomery Road to fill up my gas tank. From there, I went to grab a cup of coffee from McDonald's. After purchasing my coffee, I pulled into a vacant parking space and drank coffee while eating a serving of almonds. Silently, I prayed for a good day. Afterwards, I reached for my phone and put the school's address in it to see which direction was best to take. The directions instructed me to get on the Norwood Lateral for the quickest route. Within ten minutes, I was there.

As I entered the office, I saw a couple of familiar faces; they were both women I knew from church. I was instructed to sit in a breakroom where I heard voices over the P.A. preparing everyone for a day of school. I remember being so excited about the possibilities. I had not taught in a traditional building in over 13 years. Believe it or not, the last time I taught in a traditional setting was on the same grounds as the school I was now assigned to. During the waiting time that morning, I thought of all of the positives in the situation.

Once the announcements were completed, I was escorted to my new room that I would be sharing with another teacher. Immediately I noticed the room was nothing like my previous room. There were no windows; what was even more apparent in that moment was there was no room for me. There was no desk, no computer, no phone and no awareness that I was even a consideration at my reassigned school.

So, what did I do on my first day of my new assignment? Honestly, I sat there. I sat in my new classroom in a chair, or maybe it was a student desk. I made every effort to not be in the way of students who came in the room for instruction with their teacher.

Multiple people texted to see how it was going, but it was difficult to respond because of the bad reception. Around that time, I was studying the Book of James on the Bible app. Fortunately, my phone could connect to the app and I studied the lesson for that day. I found a blank sheet of paper and wrote down James 1:2-3 (KJV) that read, *My brethren, count it all joy when ye fall into diverse temptations; Knowing this, that the trying of your faith worketh patience.* Underneath the Scripture I wrote, "There'll be rain," making note to look up the lyrics to *It's Gonna Rain* by Kelly Price. I remember thinking in that moment, "There will be rain. Storms will come. Count it all joy."

During the last bell of the day, I went to a math class to meet the teacher and observed inclusion in a general education classroom. As the time for dismissal approached, we went back to our classroom. I asked the teacher if staff was dismissed when the students left. She assured me that our workday was over. We walked out into the hallway together and she directed me to the area where teachers entered and exited daily. I walked out the building and walked along the sidewalk to my car.

Sun shining brightly, that Monday was absolutely beautiful. I didn't even need a coat. I was thinking about how school was closed the next day due to Election Day. The Oakley Kroger was up the street and I had prepared to go grocery shopping before picking Tyler up from school. Reaching my car, I pressed the button to unlock the car and opened the trunk to get my purse.

"Today was okay. It might just work out here," I thought as I opened the door to my car. Once inside of the car, I inserted the key into the ignition and turned the key to start the car. Nothing happened. I tried again. Nothing. For some reason, my mind instructed me to press on the gas pedal. So, I pressed my foot down on the gas pedal. I could feel my foot pivoting to press down; however the pedal was not going down.

"I just need some air and I'll be fine," I said to myself. I climbed out of the car and I stood beside it with the door open. I decided to walk to the school's office, but when I arrived, it appeared dark inside. Walking back to my car, I said out loud, "What's going on with me?" But the weirdest thing happened. I was talking out loud, but it didn't sound like what I thought I was saying. Honestly, I can't tell you what I heard. I just knew it didn't make sense to me.

There was a female student sitting at the end of the walkway under a tree. Now, I was growing more concerned. I walked up to the student and asked her if she could understand what I was saying. She looked at me, like that blank stare emoticon. I realized then I needed help and quickly. *"Alex! Alex! That's who I need."*

Prior to going to the office, I had put my purse back in the trunk. I opened the trunk and grabbed my purse to get my phone cord out so I could charge my phone. I inserted the cord into the jack and the other end into the phone. I'm scared and, in my mind, the only person who could help me is my oldest son, Alex. He would know where to come to help me and I needed to call him.

I had watched a segment on a nightly news show who shared that the longer the passcode, the less likely it'll be hacked. My iPhone passcode was four words in length with the first being the longest word. I typed in the first word of the passcode. Success! Then I began to type the second word. I tried again and again, but I could not remember the rest of the passcode. *No! Wait! I need my son!* I screamed in my head.

Immediately, I unplugged the cord and put my purse back in the trunk. With my keys, my phone and my charger, I walked as quickly as I could back to the office. This time, the lights were on. Ms. Lisa, who I attend church with, was there. I tried to explain that something was physically wrong with me. She simply looked at me and immediately took me to the school nurse, who took my blood pressure. She asked me who the current president was. I won't forget what she said next.

"I'm calling an ambulance. I think she's having a stroke."

I Need You to Sit Down

Almost everything was a blur. Nothing made sense. I do remember that I did not panic nor was I frantic. Several people asked me to sit down, which I refused to do. Fear told me that sitting down would make the situation worse. So, I stood. I could hear Ms. Lisa, Nurse Brown and Ms. Barbara Cook, who I knew from when I attended my former church, talking. They were talking, but what they were saying simply fell on my confused ears.

Charades was a game I attempted to play with Ms. Lisa to inform her that I needed my purse out of the car. As I'm communicating with her, I realized that I'm making no sense in that capacity either. Sirens could be heard coming near the school. *Just great*, I am thinking. *This is my first day and the ambulance is coming for me.* I tried to find a breathable moment for all of what was happening to me to make sense.

As soon as the medics came into the office, they asked me to have a seat.

"No, I don't want to," I said as I shook my head.

They asked again and I obliged. They started asking me questions. I answered them, but my responses were met with confused faces. They asked questions again and I received the same response from my confused answers. The stretcher was brought in and they helped me on it. As we are leaving the school, the medics asked more questions.

"What's your social security number?" The medic asked.

Those were the longest single digit numbers I had probably every spoken. It literally took from the time we left the school until we entered the expressway for me to answer him.

"What's your address?" The medic asked.

I looked at him and I was so confident in my answer. However, the answer came out slowly as if I had to think of every digit and word of my address. As a matter of fact, once I got to part of my street name, I didn't know it. I simply responded, "My street name has to do with a bird that can fly."

Role Change

When I finally arrived at the emergency room at Christ Hospital, I waited with the medic for an available room. The hustle and bustle of the emergency room actually soothed me some. I just knew that I was going to get help, go home and get ready to vote the next day.

The nurses came in and asked me more questions. I noticed that they were all asking me the same questions two and three times. Now, my body was becoming exhausted. They informed me that my family was in the waiting room and they could come back in pairs. I wondered how much time had passed that my family arrived so quickly. My mom and Alex came in first. In that moment, I was truly spent, realizing that something may be wrong with me. Tyler, my youngest son, had not arrived at the hospital nor did he know anything that was going on.

Alex came in and we talked. His look was puzzling to me. Later, he would tell me that when I was asked what my birthday was, I responded with all single digits. Thinking that it was getting late, I asked Alex, "Are you going to pick up Alex from practice?"

"Momma, I am Alex," he responded, looking me directly in the eyes.

It was at that point in the hospital's emergency room that our roles changed. Yes, I am his mother and he is my oldest child. However, now, he was my caregiver, in charge of Tyler and me, and the man of the house. I had no choice in relinquishing my role. The next day, we learned that I officially had a stroke.

Black Family Reunion

My first visitors, while I was in the emergency room, were my mom and my son. What transpired after that brought me to tears. By the end of the night, everyone from my parents to my childhood friend, my siblings, my aunts, my cousins and my church family had come through. I was in that room attempting to answer the most basic questions and then people would switch out and more people would come in. I don't know what Alex did to sound the alarm, but everyone came out to see me. There were a group of people that I had to say no to and that they couldn't come in. My youngest cousins were out there, and I couldn't bear for them to see me like that. Even reflecting on it now, I would have broken completely down.

The way the story was told to me was that basically my family had shut down the waiting room. Earlier that day, my sister helped organize a career day at her school and she had a great deal of snacks leftover. So not only was my family having a reunion in the waiting room, it was complete with snacks. When my pastor showed up with my best friend, Mike, I didn't know if he needed to stay either. Mike took it way harder than I knew at the time, but he would share later how hard it was for him. Ryan and Stephanie were definitely instrumental, assuring me that even though I didn't make a whole lot of sense, they knew what I was trying to say. My cousin Lora was a ball of laughter and my aunts were in the building, too. I kept wondering, "How did all of you get here and how long have you been here?" To be honest, I had no clue as to how long I had been there myself.

I remember school had let out at 3:45 p.m., but everything after that was a blur. I was both happy to see my family and worried that they had been out too late and needed to get home for the next day. Once the nurse informed us that my room was ready, everyone prepared to go home for the night. I would discover in less than 24 hours what it meant to be overwhelmed by blessings.

Out of Sync

On November 5, 2018, I was admitted to Christ Hospital. After I was settled in my room, everyone went home and I was alone. It had been a long day and I was not offended that my family and friends had gone home. I needed the solitude. Prior to Alex leaving, he made sure my phone was charged and disengaged the passcode option. As soon as Alex left, the warmest tears fell down the side of my face.

Leaving a program and students I loved had hurt enough; and now, I'd been admitted to the hospital. The hurt was compounded. I tried to rest but as soon as I did, I would frantically wake up. My favorite verse, Romans 8:28, would come to mind. I would rattle off, "And we know that all things work together." Can I be honest? I couldn't remember *why* all things worked together. I could not remember my favorite verse in its entirety. I have loved that verse since the nineties when I went to see author Iyanla Vanzant at the Aronff Center. There, I was introduced to Angelo and Veronica who belted out the song, *All Things Work*. I went and bought their cassette tape and was led by my mom to read Romans 8 in its entirety.

Since I could not sleep, I opened the Bible app and I selected the book of Romans, Chapter 8. The Scripture appeared before me and I scrolled down to verse 28. All of the words appeared jumbled and in 3D. The words seemed to stare at me as I tried to decipher what they were. In frustration, I closed the Bible app and selected my Tidal app, where I had been steadily adding to my gospel playlist, entitled *iWorship*. I figured that if I couldn't read the Word of God, then I could sing along to some Christian music. I cued up, *My One My All* by Jesus Culture.

As I began to sing, it didn't take long to notice that I was out of sync with the music. I stopped singing and as more tears fell, I slowly fell asleep. Only this time my sleep was interrupted by a doctor waking me up. Her spirit was so gentle, and she had this beautiful long hair. I was hoping this wasn't an angelic, "touched by an angel" moment. She really made me feel comfortable until she asked me,

"What's your name?"

While I had a moment of calmness, I was now becoming frantic before the sunrise as I tried to convince her that I knew the answer.

"Wait! Wait! I know this," I said as I sat up. She sat there patiently waiting.

"I know this! I really do. Just give me a minute. In a moment of disillusionment, I worked really hard to simply say, "My name is Arlinda McKinley."

"Do you know why you're here?"

"Yes."

"Today we are taking you down for an MRI. What happened yesterday before you were brought to the hospital?"

"I had ended my first day of a new school."

More tears.

May 26, 2019

It's 7:03 p.m. I've been writing since 5:27 p.m. Today at church, my pastor spoke about dreaming big and not having a Plan B to fall back on when God is our Plan A. I received all of that message because I'm now at a point in my life where I'm totally dependent on God to protect and provide for my family and me. This is definitely a faith walk; a "Do you trust God and what He said He would do?" moment.

As I'm typing the section in regards to my playlist on my Tidal app, I remember that Tidal is live-streaming *Exodus: Music & Arts Festival*. Look at God! Not only am I working on my next book, but I have a live soundtrack to work to. Mighty are the works of your hand! Sooner or later, it will turn in my favor. All things work together.

Many or Mini
November 6, 2018

After the doctor left my room, I sat there waiting for the sun to rise completely. For the first time in years, I would not vote or be at home enjoying a day off from work. Instead I was at Christ Hospital waiting for answers and hoping for the best. Everyone on staff were so incredibly nice to me and my family. At some point, I was informed that I would have an MRI. My family sat there with me as we waited for me to go downstairs for testing. I never had an MRI before, so I had no idea what to expect.

Once I was downstairs, the nurses explained step-by-step what was going to happen. They asked me if I was claustrophobic and I honestly didn't know how to answer. Well, I imagined I answered once I was inside the MRI machine because a voice asked, "Are you okay?"

"No, I'm not," I responded. I learned that my response meant that they had to order medicine to assist with calming my nerves before they could administer the test. I guess I am claustrophobic. Once I was given medication, the process went smoothly, so much so that I didn't remember much of what had happened. What I do remember is that the doctor who had awakened me before sunrise was in my room within hours.

"We have your results back. You had a stroke," the doctor informed us. You could almost feel everyone in the room hold their breath simultaneously. She continued. "You had mini strokes in the section of your brain where speech and language is developed."

"Do you mean 'mini' as in small strokes? Or do you mean 'many' like several strokes?"

"Arlinda, you had mini strokes. That explains your slurred speech and your difficulty remembering," she calmly responded.

I thought to myself, "I am a teacher; I write, read and talk for a living. How are we going to fix this?"

"Now, we have to find out why you had a stroke. You will have a test on your heart tomorrow."

"Tomorrow? When am I going home? We have to fix this. I'm smart. I know my numbers. I don't have high blood pressure, high cholesterol and I'm not diabetic. How is this happening? You have to fix this."

"We'll have the test administered tomorrow and we'll go from there."

I was just floored and in disbelief. Alex often reminded me that I made it a point to tell all of the doctors that I was smart. Looking back, I believe that I wanted them to know that I knew my biometric data, so how was a stroke possible? Next, we were testing my heart? *My heart?!* How was my heart an issue? My heart had never been an issue. The test on Wednesday was similar to a sonogram.

Just when I thought it couldn't get any worse, it did.

Wellness Wednesday

I don't know how I was even functioning mentally at this point. I was seeing a speech therapist and an occupational therapist to assist with ensuring I could walk and take stairs independently. I was placed on a cardio diet which meant I had limited selections. Even though I had small choices, I fell in love with having a bean burger, a baked sweet potato and unsweetened applesauce for lunch. Those habits eventually became a part of my eating habits once I came home.

Today was the heart sonogram, but I'm sure that's not what it was called. I was wheeled back down to testing and the administrator explained what was about to happen. With curiosity,
I attempted to read the lady's countenance. I wanted to know if she saw anything, so I asked her what she saw. She told me that she administers the test and doctor interprets the data. Stress overcame me because something in me felt like she saw something wrong with my heart. After the procedure, I was wheeled to the end of the hallway as I sobbed uncontrollably with my head down. The orderly sat me in an area to wait for someone to take me back to my room. I remember the young lady asking me if I wanted the curtain

closed while I waited. I responded yes and sat there in despair and brokenness.

That procedure was late in the day. The nurse informed me that I would be staying another night so the doctors could read the results in the morning. By then, I had requested to the nurses to just let me know when I was being discharged. As much as I wanted to go home, I wanted to know what was going on with me. Once I had resigned to the fact that I was staying longer than I expected, I lay in my hospital bed and rested in God's arms.

Even though I had cried out that God had hurt my feelings and I was angry with Him, I stayed in my Bible app. I had my favorite Bible brought to the hospital, along with my gratitude journal and can I be honest? I had my mother bring over a Dr. Seuss book from her home that I had since I was a little girl. To prevent me from sounding like a bad karate movie, I let the music play. My hospital bed was set to an alarm and it seemed that if I even thought of moving from that bed, the blaring alarm would go off. I learned to be still as I cried, prayed and cried some more.

On Thursday morning, Alex came over really early. Somehow, we had mixed up chargers and he was bringing me a charger so that my phone's battery wouldn't die. He had taken on a huge role. After getting my youngest son up and ready for school, he had dropped him off and after coming to check on me, he was going to work. It was pretty early while I briefly chatted with my son. As he prepared to leave, as if on cue, one of the doctors who had been caring for me walked into my room.

"Good morning," said the doctor.

"Good morning," I responded.

"I have your test results. The test show that you're in the early stages of heart failure."

"Who?" I slightly yelled as I sat up. By now, my son had flopped down in the nearest chair.

"Who? I'm smart. This isn't right."

The doctor explained the data further and what the next procedure was—a TEE. TEE stands for *transesophageal echocardiography*. The procedure involves a scope going down your esophagus to view your heart. He further informed me that if there was a hole in my heart, a surgical procedure would be performed to fix it. If my heart looked good, then I would have a loop recorder implanted to monitor my heart daily.

I can't remember if Alex went to work that day; I was in such a daze. I had a stroke and now my heart was failing.

All we could do was be optimistic about the next procedure. I may not have known if my physical heart was well or not. One thing I knew for sure, my heart was broken.

I was taken to a really small room for this procedure. It was maybe three or four people in the room with me. Everyone was extremely nice as they prepared me for the test. The doctor was from Poland and I asked him how many times he had performed this procedure. The medicine to calm me was kicking in, but I vaguely remember him saying that he had performed it thousands of times. That information comforted me and it didn't take long for me to become sedated.

On the radio, I heard Whitney Houston singing. God really knew how to comfort me because I love Whitney Houston. Although I was very sad at this point, the procedure gave me a glimmer of hope. Later we would learn that my heart wasn't physically damaged. Thank God!

My cardiologist came to see me at some point to discuss implanting a loop recorder. I honestly thought that once they figured out my heart was okay that I would be free to go. But, no, not just yet.

Overwhelmed By My Blessings

Earlier, I mentioned my family's version of the "black family reunion" (BFR). By the middle of the week, I was overwhelmed by the attention and love bestowed to me. I was sad at times seeing my parents, who are getting up in age, coming to the hospital to check on me. It was supposed to be the other way around. I was supposed to be checking on them. Alex was up to my room multiple times a day and would sit with me at night before I went to sleep. Stephanie and Ryan were a force to be reckoned with. They would text or call me during the day and be there promptly in the evening with questions that demanded answers.

"What did the doctor say? What's next? You're not going back to work until after break." That last one was definitely a statement.

Enjoli would appear out of nowhere. I remember coming from an MRI and it seemed like, *Poof!* There she was.

My sister, Marlene, became my voice. I could not think beyond my current hospital room. She called my employer and those who needed to know what was going on. I don't know that I could have gotten through a lot of the employer-related issues without her. In the end, it all became too much for me to think about and process. My brother and his wife came often with cute gifts and wise words. My brother, who's the oldest of the three of us, let his protective spirit be known each time he showed up.

On any given day, my cousin Lora, my Aunt Barbara and Aunt Arlinda would be there; some with packed lunches and the latest editions of popular magazines. My Aunt Christine had also been admitted, and my cousin got her on the phone to give me words of encouragement. One Tuesday evening, everyone had left and I sat there just trying to get myself together. I would cry when I was alone since I never wanted people to see me that way. Just as the tears formed, in walked Mama Scruggs and Lady Kisha, my pastor's wife. She immediately went into prayer. I didn't know what hit me as she walked in with her swing coat flowing as she walked up to my hospital bed.

My BFF, Mike, came many times and sat with me and we laughed a lot. He really needed it because he was taking my illness really hard. I think the last to join the bunch was Scott, my former husband. He planted himself in a chair for two consecutive days. He wasn't going anywhere. Despite our trials and tribulations, he was truly with his family during our biggest crisis to date.

A Sea of Blue

Once the report came back early Friday that my heart wasn't physically damaged and I didn't need surgery, I felt a sense of relief. As a precaution, I had to have a loop recorder implanted to check for AFib. At this point, I was inundated with acronyms: TEE, MRI, AFib, and TEO. In my mind, I'm screaming that I can't keep up with all of the terms and God knows I didn't know what they meant.

Since I was a patient already at the hospital, the procedure to implant the loop recorder would be performed in my hospital room. My mom and son were there and, as only God could ordain, my former husband was there. The thing about Scott is that even after the divorce, we've managed to remain friends. I often think of the Mary J. Blige and Method Man collaboration, *You're All Need to Get By.* While we didn't work out, he's very protective over me.

As I laid in my hospital bed, there were times I just covered my entire being and silently cried as Scott and my mom discussed hints to the daily crossword puzzle and world affairs. At any moment, a doctor was going to come in and I would have to endure another stressful procedure. While each and every step was explained to me several times, it didn't assist with my anxiety concerning the situation.

"Seriously, God! I didn't do anything to deserve this. Why?" I was so hurt. I was so broken. At some point, the kindest nurses told my family that they had to leave the room; the procedure was about to begin and they could return once the procedure was complete. After my family left, way more people than I had anticipated entered my room. They all had on blue medical scrubs and they seemed to keep coming. In that moment of pain and distress, this was the prettiest sea of blue I had ever seen.

I asked the doctor performing the procedure if I could play music from my Tidal playlist. After his response, I opened my playlist and hit play. The area on the left side of my chest was cleaned and prepped for the implantation. The doctor explained every step before he did it and what I should expect as a result of it. To keep the cleaned area sanitized, there was a medical assistant who placed a towel on a rack and let it hang slightly past my chin to prevent my breath from contaminating the sanitized site.

Almost on cue, *You Know My Name* by Tasha Cobbs-Leonard and Jimi Cravity began to play. Next, *King of Glory* by Todd Dulaney played. The nurses consistently asked if I was okay. That was so comforting to me. When the doctor was ready to make the incision, *My One My All* by Jesus Culture featuring Chris McClarney was playing. For the first time in days, I could actually sing along. As the incision was made and the loop recorder was implanted, I sang, "No other hope, no other love, my one my all Jesus. No other God, no one all above; you're all I want."

I drifted back to when my niece, Ryan, and I attended Woman Evolve Conference in Denver, Colorado over the summer. That was my first time hearing the song and now it was one of the songs that was bringing me through a rough time. So much had changed in my life; reassignment, new location and now my medical condition. Throughout all of it, all that I wanted was Jesus. I wanted His love, His presence and in this instance, Jesus was truly more than everything to me.

When the procedure was complete, the doctor paired my loop recorder to the monitor that I would be taking home with me. I've paired several things in my life—headphones and wireless speakers—but pairing a device to monitor my heart was definitely a first. As the sea of blue left out of my hospital room, the nurses on the floor came in and sat with me. They gently told me that I was being discharged. It was now time to go home to the place where I wanted to go so badly on that past Monday evening while I sat in the emergency room. I was finally going to that place that I loved, where I found peace. My sanctuary.

My Sanctuary

My home has always been affectionately called my sanctuary. It's my place of refuge. It's where I find peace and serenity. I was more than elated to walk through the front door, to the excited barks of our dog on that cold November night. Immediately, I was ushered to my bed by Alex. Moments later, Stephanie, Ryan and Calvin came to visit. It was a surreal moment, whereas I believe I was in a trance for a while. That week had been huge in my life and in exactly one week, I would be turning 49. I generally planned to go to my favorite restaurant, The Capital Grille. However, after my health scare, I hadn't even thought about celebrating my birthday. Especially after learning that I had to have an MRI administered on my heart that next Monday.

After everyone went home, I decided to do the only thing that I could do and that was to turn in for the night. The best part of this idea is that I would be sleeping in my own bed, under my own comforters, with the calming sounds of trains traveling to and fro. I tend to find peace in what others would call "noise." Therefore, for me the sounds of the trains are soothing to my soul.

As Alex organized my prescriptions and set up my loop recorder monitor, I told him that he had done so much that week and for my return home, I needed him to go out with his friends and be his 25-year-old self. I ensured him that I would be okay, but prior to him leaving, he made sure that my passcode was disabled on my phone. In days to come, Ryan would instruct me to put my phone on "Do Not Disturb" during the day so I could rest. During my period of rest, I couldn't cook or drive for weeks. That home that I loved so much was the place where I'd heal and turn to God in deciding my next moves. My pastor always tells us to make our next move our best move. Now, I was given the time to figure out just what my next move would be.

On November 10th, I made my first Instagram post, which was a repost from @realtalkkim. The post read, "God said, I'm restoring you as if it never happened." I so believed that in my heart, that God was going to use this experience to bless and be a light for others. Even months later, I still believe this.

Happy Birthday

I hadn't planned to celebrate my birthday, but Alex insisted on it. He made reservations for J. Alexander's Redland for us. Alex told me that on that night, it would just be us—my two pumpkins and me. My sons just wanted "Mommy-Son" time. As a mom, it was so difficult to focus on my healing knowing they were hurting, too. Alex was being the strong one, but not really taking the time to understand how he was doing personally; and then, Tyler's grades began to plummet. My prayer life definitely shifted. My family was struggling, and I needed God to answer some prayers.

Since being discharged, I made it a point to dress cute daily for me. I needed to look good, even if I didn't feel good. On my birthday night, I made extra effort. I put on a really cute black, asymmetrical, one-sleeved dress I had purchased from Lane Bryant to wear to a wedding in the spring, along with a pair of black boots. I remember Alex asking, "What the Mary J. Blige is going on here?" We both laughed really hard, something that hadn't been done in a while.

At the restaurant, my sons gifted me a beautiful bouquet of flowers and the newly released, *Becoming*, by our forever First Lady Michelle Obama. They noticed that while

I was in the hospital and after coming home that I gravitated to reading and watching television programing about Mrs. Obama. Little did I know that, in those moments, I was becoming who God intended me to be all along.

Dinner was over and as we left the restaurant, a group of women walked past me. One lady in particular reached out and asked for my flowers jokingly. I looked at my sons and asked them if it was okay to give them to her. He affirmed and I walked up to her and handed my beautiful bouquet to her. She became a little emotional and told me that things had been hard for her lately and the flowers made her feel better. I shared with her my testimony and we hugged. A lady with the group told me that it was her husband's birthday and as he entered the restaurant, my family wished him a happy birthday, too. It's just like God to be so amazing that while my sons celebrated me, I, in return, would bless and comfort another person.

It's Not Supposed to Be This Way

One day, I remember opening my email and seeing an advertisement for Lysa TerKeurst's latest book, *It's Not Supposed to Be This Way*. I immediately rolled my eyes up to the ceiling and said, "Yeah, I probably need this book because it's really not supposed to be this way." Approximately year ago, I read *Uninvited* by Lysa TerKeurst and so I knew that I would purchase her latest release.

The Saturday after my birthday, my friend from church, Kerrence, came over so that we could talk about my medicine and changing my eating habits. During our girlfriend-wellness visit, we had tea time as we discussed everything. She explained the medicines and some of their side effects, and what I could eat now that my cardiologist had placed me on a low sodium diet. My goal was to manage 1500mg or less of sodium a day; therefore, we came up with a plan for me to eat similar to how I ate in the hospital.

As we were talking, Alex brought me the mail, which included a bulky package. I opened it and was in utter shock when I saw the book from my email, *It's Not Supposed To Be This Way*. Surprised was a complete understatement. Honestly, I wondered, *Did I order this book and not remember that I did?* Upon Kerrence leaving, I contacted the shipper and learned that no name was associated with the shipment. For the rest of the day, I was consumed with whether I ordered the book and if the stroke had a deeper impact than I assumed. And if I didn't order it, who did?

Nevertheless, I began reading the book that night. However, reading was a struggle which would be addressed in speech therapy. Yes, the intervention specialist needed speech therapy! But after reading a few paragraphs, I prayed to God to help me figure out who sent me the book. After praying, a name dropped in my spirit...Quiera. It was Dr. Quiera Lige who would soon be Mrs. Quiera Banks. I sent her a text and she confirmed that when she saw the book, she felt it would help with my healing. Look at God!

MRI

On the Monday after my release, I was scheduled for an MRI. With the diagnosis of my heart operating at early stages of heart failure, I was told that this would give the doctor more information about my heart. I understood the test was necessary, but I didn't want to return to the hospital so soon. My thoughts were very direct. This test could have been taken again while I was admitted to the hospital.

Once I got dressed in my hospital gown, I talked to a nurse regarding my concerns about the last MRI experience. I asked her about medicine to assist with my claustrophobia. She told me that I had to let my doctor know and he would have prescribed something for me prior to the test. How would I have known that? There was no checklist or instructions provided.

Now, I was nervous and anxious, knowing that I had to go through the process without medicinal assistance. Once we arrived to the procedure room, the nurse set everything up and explained what was going to happen. The test would be about an hour and I don't know how I was going to get through it, but I had to. She asked me what type of music I wanted to listen to and I responded, "gospel music."

Once inside the MRI machine, besides the close fit of the machine, I remembered the thick gray strip that ran down the middle of the machine. I kept my eyes focused on that line and followed all of the instructions given to me.

"Breathe in. Hold it for a various number of seconds. Exhale."

This went on which seemed like eternity. As the music played through the machine, I was thinking and hoping the music would help. I had no idea which artist was singing, but he started belting out, "The grave is underneath me." I rolled my eyes and thought, *That is the last thing I wanted to hear about in this machine was the grave.*

If I ever need another MRI, I'm going to request rap music.

Speech Therapy

Attending speech therapy was a challenge in the beginning. The therapist would challenge me with various puzzles and activities. The first couple of weeks, I would leave with a terribly bad headache, go home and go directly to sleep. As an educator, I have collaborated with speech therapists for years and now the intervention specialist needed speech therapy. A big takeaway was that it dismantled my perception of speech. I had to relearn how to organize my thoughts and take on tasks that made sense to me without stressing me out.

Since I was a little girl, I've always been an avid reader and writer. But now, I had to chunk in time each day to get used to doing those things again. Printed text was overwhelming, and writing out my thoughts proved to be challenging. Sometimes, I would write something and reread it and my heart sank at the numerous grammatical errors. A couple of days after being in the hospital, my sister asked me to reread a text I sent to her. After looking at the text, I looked at other texts I had sent. They all had errors, and some made no sense at all. Can you imagine how frustrating that was for me? Not only was I a writer, blogger and teacher, but I taught English! I loved social media, but I was at a point where I didn't want to write because it was too stressful.

My therapist picked up on so much about me being hesitant to open up to her. She encouraged me to start typing and writing again. Outside of writing, she even had to assist me with going back to church and to the grocery store. I was experiencing overstimulation. If a location had too many people, loud noise and bright lights, I was not a fan. The first Sunday I went back to church, I wondered if I would come back. It was too much. Also, it didn't help that I sat in front of the drummer either. When church was over, I wanted to go straight home. The grocery store with its too many bright lights and grocery aisles was my Goliath. For months, I went directly to what I needed and got out of there.

The outgoing independent woman that would go from work, to picking up her son at school, to the grocery store, back home to cook and off to a meeting or a class had been sidelined. I wanted so badly to get back to my daily routine and that became extremely important to me. During a session, my therapist had a gentle moment with me. It was almost as if she was spiritually holding my hand as she said, "Arlinda, I don't think it has hit you yet; the magnitude of what has happened to you."

I asked her to elaborate to get a better understanding.

She went on to tell me that it could have been worse. I guess I was still oblivious, because I asked, "How?"

Very patiently, her gentle spirit answered my question.

All of my energy was relative to getting back to normal, not realizing that if more time had passed on November 5th with no treatment, I could have had a very different outcome. Moreover, inclusive of not being able to be here to share my story with you.

All Call

One thing that I strived for after coming home was independence. The first couple of weeks I didn't cook for myself. I learned that my nephew cooked the best bean burgers. I felt as if I had short order cooks living in my home. I couldn't drive to my various appointments. Stephanie, my childhood friend of over 30 years, took me to my doctor appointments. We laughed a lot and listened to music trying to decide if twerking was something I should be trying to do. I wanted so desperately to get back to normal and be independent again. Oftentimes, I felt like I was a burden to people. But once I was cleared to drive, I was super excited.

One day, I woke up and my blood pressure dropped drastically, and I was extremely tired. So, I made an appointment to see my doctor. I called or texted Alex that I was going to the doctor but I don't think I told him what for. While at the doctor's office, I didn't pay much attention to my phone because I felt so tired. I was more occupied with finding out *why* I felt the way I did. What I learned that day was that my prescription needed to be lowered and that my oldest son needed to know my every movement until further notice.

When I arrived home, I noticed my son's car was there, but didn't think anything of it. I walked into the living room to the concerned faces of my son, my nephew and his girlfriend, and my brother and sister-in-law. Quite surprised, I asked them why was everyone at my house. They all looked at me like I was crazy.

Then Alex, in a very stern tone says, "Mama! You didn't answer my call. I thought something happened."

He had made one call and they all showed up. Their concern for my health quickly turned to their concern for me to understand how my health scares were impacting my entire family.

New Year's Eve

Generally, on New Year's Eve, I sulked because it was my wedding day. It was always a reminder of the marriage that failed. Somehow, this New Year's Eve of 2018 was a tad different. On this day, my sister and my two sons sat with me in a small patient room at UC's Neurology Department. As we sat there, the tone was as solemn as the gray skies and dreary day.

It's still mind boggling that I was waiting to see a neurologist. Can I pause for a moment and share that up until sometime in November, I had no clue how to spell neurologist? I just relied on my Webster app to spell it correctly. I guess it's just one of those words that I never thought I would use regularly. I would start with the letter "n" and could not decide if the next two letters were "eu" or "ue." Now I can write the words *neurologist* and *neurology* with ease.

The doctor entered the small room filled with my family. She sat down on the chair next to the computer and looked over my medical information and asked the question that every doctor had asked me.

"What was going on the day that you had a stroke?"

"Can I go back to the prior week?" I asked.

She simply responded, "Start where you think it's relevant."

I sat on the patient bed and looked at my reflection in the window. I was as gloomy as the weather. I began my story with a day designed for costumes and trick or treat, Halloween.

She's Back

On January 8, 2019, I returned to work. I had always wondered how I would feel going back to the place where I had a stroke. To make the drive easier, I went to Tidal and turned on *My One My All* by Jesus Culture. Yes, tears fell. They always do. I rode to work with a sense of peace knowing that God works all things together for good. I doubt some things, but I don't doubt that God took me on this journey so that I may be a light of hope for others; therefore, God gets the glory.

When I went in to work that day, I had tokens of gratitude for Ms. Lisa and Nurse Brown. The day before I was out shopping, and I saw two ceramic angels. That's what those two women were to me on November 5th. I'm so thankful for everyone who stood in the gap for me. Those who prayed when I couldn't because of the shock of it all. Those who sat with me, talked for me, drove me to appointments, cooked for us, gifted us and made sure my family was taken care of.

I've grown up hearing clichés in the church. One being, "He's a doctor in a sick room." You really don't fully understand that until you need Him to be a doctor in *your* sick room.

May 27, 2019

After reading this over, I am most amazed that I really thought that coming back to work and getting back to "normal" was going to be the end of the story as if this was a fairy tale ending. Nothing could be farther from the truth. Going back to work only proved to incite more diagnoses, antidepressants and therapy for anxiety and PTSD.

Headaches

One of the side effects of my stroke were the headaches. Not only did they hurt immensely, but they were turning into the biggest nuisance. I could go two or three days without having one and the intense pain would show up. It was hard to read long passages. Bright lights and rooms full of people overwhelmed me. Just thinking about everything triggered a headache.

I was told that it wasn't uncommon for people to experience headaches after having a stroke. It was suggested that I drink more water and go for a walk at the onset of a headache. Taking medicine was not an option for me because I was bothered that I was already taking several medications. I just didn't want to see or have to ingest another pill.

At one of my latest visits, my doctor suggested two things: First, to take ibuprofen with Gatorade; and second, a prescription for headaches. I decided to try the prescription, even though I didn't want to. My doctor informed me that it would help with my headaches and sleep. I hadn't been doing well in the area of sleep since having a stroke either. The thought of no headaches and a good night's sleep was extremely inviting and the deciding factors to try the medication.

That night as I prepared for bed, I read the information about the prescription. I opened up the trifold brochure and one word caught my eye. A word that I had heard recently but didn't really consider. That word was *antidepressant*. Minutes prior, I thought about starting the prescription on the weekend, but then I read over the list of symptoms that the medicine addressed. Since I needed to sleep for the headaches to stop and for the anxiety to subside, I decided to begin that night.

Not only did I sleep well, but I felt a little better the next day. For the first time in months, I didn't acknowledge the loop recorder monitor beside my bed. Yes, faith without works is dead. Just maybe, seeking medical care is part of the "works."

Therapy

"For God hath not given us the spirit of fear; but of power, and of love, and of a sound mind."
2 Timothy 1:7 (KJV)

By mid-November, I knew I needed more supports in place than what I had. In the African American community, we often don't seek medical assistance for mental health-related issues. It's such a stigma that many are trying to address, especially with the increasing numbers in youth suicide. I picked up the phone and made an appointment because not only was I not handling everything well, some things I wasn't even handling them at all. During our session my therapist posed a pivotal question.

"Did God or Pharaoh tell you to go to your new assignment?" the therapist asked.

"I don't know. You mean like Pharaoh who Moses told to let his people go?" I responded.

Silence.

"Arlinda, you've been teaching for 16 years. You've gone through sweatless doors for years and now your foundation is shaking," the therapist offered. "You've had a pattern for not speaking up for yourself. You limit your voice with people who don't treat you well. Think about this. The stroke impacted the part of your brain that impacts your voice. The voice that you are hesitant to use."

I had never considered the impact of my voice, I thought.

"Maybe this is God getting your attention. Maybe you are no longer an intervention specialist. You do write books, right? Maybe you're an author now."

I had never considered not being a teacher. I sat there and let her words sink in. Not teach? Author?

The therapist turned to her calendar to set the next appointment. "Is March 8th good for you?"

"Yes," I replied.

I left her office and walked down the tree-lined streets and thought about our conversation. She was right about my career with the district. Even when I first came to the district I always had assignments, whether they were day to day assignments or long-term substitute positions. Long-term positions were assignments that lasted 21 days or more. Once I earned my special education licensure, I went on to study for my administration certification. I felt like I was on track to move up in my career. For her to tell me to consider that I was no longer an intervention specialist hit me hard. I loved what I did and my students.

I had to be really honest. While I truly loved my job. I wasn't completely happy there. In some ways, I was actually bored. It was maybe September or October when I looked out the window in my classroom and said, "There has to be more to my life than this." I needed an outlet to both serve children and be creative and I wasn't able to do that in my former position. On ride home I kept hearing my therapist's words and thought, "What am I supposed to do? I needed my job for income and insurance. I had to somehow at least finish out the school year and then spend the summer considering my options.

Primary Meltdown 25

I had only been back to work for three weeks and I promise you, I had not made it one full week. I'd go to sleep each night thinking, *I can do this. I have to get back to normal. Whatever normal is.* Yet, something didn't feel right.

The first week that I returned, I worked half days. Still, there was no place for me at that school. Maybe complaining about not having teacher essentials was really a sign of something else. On November 5th when I arrived there, I didn't have a desk, a computer, a phone or a class list. Isn't that "Teacher Essentials 101"? I came back months later and I did have a phone. But, it was on the table where students worked. There were no extra desks in the building and if I needed to use a computer, I could share with the teacher I was sharing the room with.

I had been listening a lot to Jonathan McReynolds' latest CD, *Make Room,* and came to the conclusion that still there was no room for me there. Heck! I even had to send an email requesting a key for the classroom. Frustration was setting in. In three weeks' time, I was diagnosed with depression and prescribed anti-depressants. Later, I was diagnosed with anxiety and couldn't sleep well. My primary care doctor suggested that I seek other medical care to assist with my mental health, which was now plummeting at a rapid rate. I experienced instability at work and later learned that I was having negative reactions by returning to the place where I had a stroke.

What I tried to convey to everyone is at that point in my life, I needed consistency. I needed to know that each day I had a set schedule and class list. Instead, I was used as a substitute teacher with various groups of students who not only did I not know, but I also had no clue what they were studying. There were parts of me screaming out that I needed help and I needed it badly. It seemed the more I voiced my need for structure, the worse it got.

On January 23rd and 24th, I was off work t doctor's appointments. I started therapy and the therapist gave me some tools to assist me in getting through the school days. I remember coming back to school that Friday and someone saying, "I'm sorry Ms. McKinley, but we are short of a lot of staff today. We need you to sub for 7th grade math."

The day started out well, but as the day went on, it became unbearable. I honestly tried to hold it together. But, when the students returned from lunch, I picked up the phone and told the secretary that I had to leave. Relief was sent to the classroom, I picked up my things and left. As I was walking to the exit, I was stopped by a teacher and we had a conversation. He was actually one of the nicest things about my experience there. I shared with him that being in that building subbing all the time and feeling disregarded was too much for me and that I wasn't coming back. I loved teaching, and I loved the children. I even loved math. But that setting was no longer healthy for me.

When I share this with people, I tell them I did a "Colin Kaepernick" and took a knee. At that point, I had to make a stance. I was reassigned because my school's numbers were low, and this school had a high number of junior high school students. I do understand they needed another teacher for well-deserving students. I was sent there for that reason, but all I did was substitute teach. When I wasn't substituting, I either sat in a room or I went and asked other teachers if they needed help. Even as I sit here now and write this book, my chest hurts as I think about that experience. It stills takes my anxiety to another level.

It was shared with me that my colleagues were informed that I was stressed and struggling when I arrived at the new school because I hadn't been in a general education building in years. That was so far from the truth since I was never given an opportunity to use my skillset or educational background at my new position. In a nontraditional setting, I had taught students who, at times, were on parole or in jail waiting to be placed in prison. I had taught overaged students who were credit deficient for over a decade, many who came from unimaginable circumstances. So, to say that I was struggling for that reason provides a false narrative of who I am. I was just seen as another body in the building to help substitute and fill in. I've always been the teacher who wanted to get boys of color off the school-to-prison pipeline. I've never shied away from that passion of helping students be their best selves.

On the 25th of January, I felt completely unwelcomed and unwanted. It showed up in my physical health in November when I had the stroke and now, it was rearing its ugly head in my mental health. I chose to leave that place, leaving behind hurtful memories. I also remembered that, prior to working there, I was not on any prescription medications and I didn't have any medical diagnoses nor had I experienced having any meltdowns.

There were two phrases that I remember voicing constantly and clearly during those three weeks, "This is too much for me" and "I'm not going back there." I knew that if that school was my only option, then I had no options.

Solange

As I scrolled through Instagram one day, I read that Solange had dropped a new release and there was a video on iTunes. There was something that called me to watch the video and I watched it once. Then again and again. It reminded me of a futuristic scene from *The Wiz* and I was very drawn to it. I went online to listen and for days I couldn't get past listening to tracks one through nine. I must admit that I was hooked. *Stay Flo* easily became my song. I loved it and danced to it every time I heard it.

Within the next two weeks, I let the entire project play. The entire album brought me such peace and comfort in my time of darkness and uncertainty. *When I Get Home* takes me to a place of peace and serenity. When I listened to each song, I felt as if I was surrounded by peaceful flowing water. There were some nights that I turned it on before I went to sleep and set it to repeat, allowing it to play all night long. On days that I was really struggling, I played *Dreams* and reminded myself of all the dreams I had as a little girl and how they were sidetracked by heartbreak or lack of self-confidence. "Those dreams come a long way," sings Solange.

Often, I've had conversations about why I love this project so much. I think the trauma that I've experienced sat me down to be open to the beautiful body of work, *When I Get Home.* If Iyanla Vanzant is my auntie in my head, then Solange is the play cousin that I've yet to meet. I need her to know that while she was growing through her healing, she created one of my favorite albums and God used her gift to assist me through a difficult time.

The questions I'm asked often are, "Arlinda, what are you going to do now? What's next?"

I found my answer while listening to the song *Binz:* "Imma get back on my feet. Give me a minute."

I Choose Joy

On March 8th, I woke up and prepared for my day. As with every payday, I checked my checking account. However, on this day, I didn't get paid by my employer. I decided that in that moment I wasn't going to get upset. God had been good to me thus far and there was no reason to think that He didn't have that under control either. Weeks prior, my parents purchased new furniture and I asked if I could have my grandmother's recliner. My grandmother had passed several years ago, and I couldn't let them get rid of her chair.

When the chair arrived at our home, we had no idea where we would put it. Alex's idea was to place it next to our ottoman that sat in the middle of the room. I told him that it didn't make sense, although to this day that is where I sit to watch Sports Center in the morning with my Greek yogurt or steel-cut oatmeal. I was sitting in that chair upon realizing that I had no pay and a therapy appointment in an hour. God spoke to me as I sat there.

"If you had to go back to where you were reassigned in order to get paid today, would you go?"

My immediate response was, "No; I choose joy!"

Joy was what I felt now. I had become a beautiful butterfly who was free flowing in the direction that God had destined for me. No longer was I allowing people to treat me any kind of way. I was flowing in a different direction; therefore, *this* would not affect me. I sat there and I had a full understanding that my time with my employer was coming to an end.

"I'm proud of how you're handling this," said my therapist.

"Me too. It's hard to believe sometimes. I'm not mad anymore. Just clear," I responded. "I have decided that if this isn't resolved and I'm not paid during the next pay period, I'm resigning from the district."

"Really? That's huge Arlinda. I think back to when I started seeing you years ago and how you've grown. Do you know what it means if you resign?" She asked.

"That I have to find another job?" I inquired.

"No, it means that you break a generational curse over your life," she declared.

"Really? Me? I'm breaking a generational curse?" I asked excitedly.

"How old will you be this year?" she asked.

"Fifty," I responded.

"Five is the number of grace. You're now walking in God's grace," she told me after looking on her computer.

"And today is the eighth of March. Eight is new beginnings and three is the number of the trinity," I said.

"Today is also International Women's Day," she chimed in.

I left therapy that day knowing that everything was going to be okay and that everything was unfolding as it was supposed to. I called my mother once I got into my car and told her about the session. My mom became quiet and a short time later told me that today was my great-grandmother's birthday.

I learn it's my great-grandmother's birthday on the day that I'm informed that I'm breaking a generational curse. My great-grandmother's name was Ura. I've been told that when my grandmother gave birth to my aunt, they used a combination of Ura and Linda to come up with the name Arlinda. That name was passed to me. I'm sure that she would have wanted me to break a generational curse and go forth to be the woman that she had prayed for.

At this point, I knew I had to resign. I just wasn't sure if I would actually go through with it.

I didn't get paid the next pay period either. I sat on the couch, still disappointed and upset. But God was there with me at each step. I knew that I had to let go, that I couldn't go another day being employed with a company that knowingly withheld my pay, expecting me to pay for health insurance out of pocket because of a decision that they had made. The level of trust that I had with my employer was fading to black.

It was simply time for me to leave, to be at peace and to truly heal from the stroke and everything that transpired afterwards.

Chapter Closed ~ April 11, 2019

I woke up that morning with scents of peppermint and lavender from my oil diffuser and YouTube playing some 528 MHz heart chakra music. I learned about healing music while attending a "Relax and Restore" series. The facilitator talked to us about healing music and how certain frequencies have healing qualities. She even shared that certain frequencies can change your DNA. 528 MHz in one such frequency. She challenged us to type in 528 MHz in the YouTube search bar and listen. Sadaqa, our facilitator was so informative and caring over everyone in attendance as we were introduced to information that we'd never heard of.

Besides healing music, she introduced many of us to *chakras*. Chakras are seven centers in our body where energy flows through: root chakra, sacral chakra, solar chakra, heart chakra, throat chakra, third eye chakra and the crown chakra. She even gave each of us a beautiful Chakra bracelet that also included clay beads. The clay beads could be used as a diffuser by adding essential oils.

I read my plans in the Bible App and decided that I was going to implement a "speak well/eat well" mindset. Career wise, I was spent and just beyond frustrated. I had been with my employer for nearly 17 years and once I had a stroke, it seemed as if I was punished because of it. For one entire month, I went without being paid and no explanation as to why. Now the union, who rescinded my resignation, was fighting for my sick time, the same sick time I was supposed to be paid when it was suggested that I go out on medical leave by Human Resources. So now, the powers that be were trying to decide if I should receive my sick pay. I wanted to wait it out and let their decision become the end of it all. That's at least what I thought.

By 9:00 that morning, I called my union representative, who was an extreme blessing to my family and me. I told her that I didn't want her to fight any more for the promised advanced sick days—the same advanced sick days that Human Resources instructed her to request for me and she had done exactly that. I honestly just wanted this to be over and I wanted my resignation to go through the minutes of the board. I did feel as though I had been treated unfairly, especially after being approved for FMLA (Family and Medical Leave Act). Now, I needed that door in my life to close to move on with my life.

There were several people who were disappointed with my decision. They felt that I should have stayed and fought more. I totally understood and it wasn't that I didn't have it in me to fight. I'd just rather focus my energy on maintaining my post-stroke headaches, making sure my blood pressure didn't go drastically up from stress or drastically low from being on blood pressure medicine. I wanted to remain calm so that my loop recorder didn't download data to my cardiologist that would have resulted in calls from his office. I also wanted to focus on the sharp pains on my right side that occurred because my brain didn't register that when I was cold, that I was cold. Instead, it registered as pain.

So I asked myself this: *Do I want to sit and fight the same people who gave me two days to pack 10 years of my life? No. Do I want to sit and fight the people who made a leave plan for me and didn't honor it? No. Do I want to fight the same group of people who didn't pay me for an entire month, nor respond to any correspondence in regard to this matter? No.*

This battle was not mine to fight; it was the Lord's. The very best thing that I could do for myself was to be like the character in *Frozen* and let it go. I had to let go in order to heal, to grow and to be prepared for what God had next for me. For only God truly knows what's best for me as Jeremiah 29:11 tell us this. On that same day, I reposted an Instagram post by @womenbychoice that stated, "And when God opens this next door, you're going to understand why the enemy fought you so hard."

In October of 2016, I was introduced to the ministry of Pastor Michael Beckwith via Super Soul Sunday, which airs on OWN. He talked about this idea of "unfolding" and being vibrational. My body was trying to tell me something with the stroke, the depression and the anxiety. I was unfolding. My illnesses were pushing me to make the decision to move onto what God had next for me.

Those past five months were incredibly hard for me. The disregard for my being had been challenging. Often, I went to God and simply said, "What did I do to these people? It seemed to be one problem after another."

God never responded. He just listened to my rants. Then a phrase by Pastor Beckwith came to mind, "Pain pushes until vision pulls."

Without me realizing it, being vibrational, I was being crushed for God's planned purpose for my life. Although it hurt and at times I was under incredible stress on the journey, I knew that I couldn't go back to an environment that didn't support the amazing person that I am.

So, what's next for Arlinda? Only God knows. I have several unique opportunities to assist people in growing their business by working for them in an administrative capacity. Both would allow me to use my administrative skills and my education background. All of the requests were totally unexpected, and I believe God sent them to me on purpose.

At 6:33 a.m. nearly every morning, for many years, I recite Matthew 6:33, The Prayer of Jabez and The Serenity

Prayer. I'll continue to ask God to bless me indeed, for wisdom on things that I can and cannot change and to diligently seek Him and His righteousness.

I wrote this journal while listening to Open My Heart by Yolanda Adams & Let Me Touch You by Kirk Franklin.

Tethered

The struggle of this journey has forced me to make some pretty huge decisions which were difficult. Carefully, I weighed them several times on a daily basis, considering the possibilities. Can I be honest? People were simply treating me badly in their tones and responses. Now, I'm not perfect and I fall short daily. I believe in having grace and compassion for others, even though I didn't feel that at all from others. I felt lonely, disregarded, unwelcomed and uninvited. People were not kind, and many showed that they couldn't care less about my physical or mental health. Each time I walked through the doors at work, every time I had received a voicemail or email in response to my growing concerns, I felt the disregard and animosity.

It was so painful that I brought it up in therapy, to my pastor and even in my time alone with God. I constantly expressed my concerns and how it made me feel. I never felt that way in my life and to feel it every day at my place of employment was taking a toll on me. One day, God spoke to me about the matter. He told me that what I was experiencing was not how He treats me or how He wants anyone to treat me. He said, "I no longer want you tethered to places or people who don't see you and value you as I do." *Tethered?*

I immediately thought about the childhood game of tether ball. The only thing that I know for sure about the game is that no matter how hard you hit the ball, the only thing it would do was wrap around the pole. The ball never left the rope and the rope never left the ball. Well, it would leave the pole if the rope was frayed or if someone physically cut the rope from the pole. Once the rope was cut from the pole, the ball was free—free from people hitting it and from being attached to a pole that was stationary. Cutting the ball from the rope freed the ball to be used for other purposes.

God was severing the ties. He was cutting me from the rope. In those moments, all I could think of was my teaching career of almost 20 years, my salary, my medical insurance and the stability of my family. I was focused on things that seemed minute to God. He owns cattle on a thousand hills, and the fullness of the earth is His (Psalm 50:10). Surely, He would see me through this, too. I've found that God was focused on something bigger. God was focused on something oblivious to me: My freedom to be at peace to be exactly who He had created me to be.

"Arlinda, maybe you're no longer an intervention specialist. Maybe you're now a full-time writer."

I thought back many times to that therapy session on March 8th, the first time I didn't get paid because I was, unknowingly, coded at work leave with no pay. That session was a pivotal moment for me and then May 25th came, a little over a month after I resigned from my former employer. My pastor, Dr. Michael Scruggs, preached a sermon entitled, "No Limits" from Ephesians 3:20. Normally, I don't sit on the front row at church. But, this particular morning, I did, and God had my undivided attention. My pastor talked about taking the limits off. He discussed how God never created you to be ordinary and God has so much more for you. He told us that the stuff you're tripping on is nothing to God.

Pastor Mike was on a roll that morning. Near the end of the sermon, he spoke on a topic that shifted everything for me. He said two words: *Tether ball*. I saw everything come together in that moment. This entire journey wasn't about all of the things that I believed it to be. This was about God trusting me to burn the plow of my Plan B and fully trusting my Plan A. God is my Plan A. My Plan B had become my comfort; the place where I knew that I had the things I needed. God wanted more for me, to release the aspect of having a comfort zone and venture out to uncharted waters and be a light for Him.

The sermon was confirmation of what God was doing in my life. To some people, my decision seemed foolish. Questions were asked.

"What about Tyler? You still have to raise him."

"How are you going to pay your bills?"

"What about your mortgage?"

I remember responding to someone by saying, "I rep God well. He loves me. He always takes care of me. If He told me to leave my employer, He's not going to have me looking stupid." That was an honest statement from the depth of my heart. As my pastor said, "Faith is the willingness to look foolish."

And without faith, it's impossible to please God... (Hebrews 11:6)

Final Fridays ~ Do It Scared

With everything going on, I sat down one Sunday evening and talked to Lady Kisha, our first lady at Light of the World Church. We were just talking about everything that I was going through and how excited she was about what God was doing in my life. She so gently told me that I would now lead our Women's Ministry. We talked about how I had been running from it. Now, I could see that I was finally running *to* it, because I didn't fight it.

Our Women's Ministry meets on the final Friday of each month to study, pray and fellowship. For several years, my friend Enjoli and I had planned and facilitated the meeting together, but they were moving her to a different area solely and now I had to do it solo for our church. After more people learned that I had resigned from my job, they would ask me, "What are you going to do now?"

Now, I would always say, "I'm going into ministry full-time and do what God wants me to do." I guess I was finally manifesting a truth in my life.

At church, I had been pleasantly pleased to be in the background and now that was about to change. Truthfully, I was scared. I was scared that I would get super nervous and not know what I was doing. I was scared that people would look at me with a bunch of blank stares. I was scared that I wasn't good enough, cute enough or smart enough. I watch a lot of pastors online and when they speak on fear, they all have the same message:

"Do it scared. Do it afraid. Do it unsure. Just do it. You'll never know that you can't do something until you actually bust a faith move." And I did!

On April 26, 2019, I facilitated "Final Fridays" by myself. The blueprint had been created weeks in advance. The study was based on two things, Kierra Sheard's song *Reppin' My God* and Esther 2:13. It was creatively entitled, "Who Said I Can't Be Fly?" Not only did we talk about Chapter 2 of the Book of Esther, but we also discussed being stylish and saved. Our meeting was complete with an impromptu fashion show with participants from the Bible study. I was scared that night, but I did it anyway. Afterwards, my adrenalin was high. I couldn't eat or sleep until I had created a Facebook event page for the next session, where we would discuss what the Bible says about self-care.

All those gifts that I had been blessed with—being an avid researcher, a creative soul with a desire to share with women—are the things that assist them being their best selves. A pseudo-technology geek was now being used for God's glory. I was free to be me, finally!

Diligently

During my first medical leave, several people encouraged me to write a book and I brushed it aside, well the writing part anyway. However, the title was etched in my mind. The book would be entitled *Speechless*. I chose that title because that's what I was feeling towards God. Not only were my feelings hurt, but having a stroke and the possibility of heart failure had rendered me speechless. I just couldn't believe God. I was losing weight and keeping up with my biometrics and I had a stroke. I was at such a loss with God.

Even in those moments, I stayed in God's Word, attended church and read the Bible and Bible plans. I had a close circle of friends who prayed for me and with me. I listened to gospel and Christian music. I listened to my favorite pastors often: Pastor Jamal Harrison Bryant, Pastor Sarah Jakes-Roberts and Pastor TD Jakes. I relived Woman Evolve 2018 and watched Woman Thou Art Loosed 2019 via the app. I listened to my auntie (in my head), Iyanla Vanzant, to try and fix my life on Saturday evenings. I was introduced to the awesome Dr. Thema Bryant-Davis while she helped Chad and Michelle. There was a show on OWN entitled "Chad Loves Michelle." Chad, who is a minister, was engaged to Michelle, a former member of Destiny's Child. Dr. Thema was their therapist. Online, I was following heavy hitters for

Christos, @brokentopeace, @jolynne_whittaker_official, @neechyofficial, @curtricelwilliams and @kristylyles. I was trying to get everything I could to help me through this dark time.

Going out on my second medical leave was totally different from the first one. I was at peace and I wanted to know more about God, His love and His plans for me. I was sitting in my living room and I said, "Without faith, it's impossible to please God." I thought that was the actual Scripture. I go online to find the Scripture to read it in its entirety. I was directed to Hebrews 11:6 and I read the Scripture out loud.

"And without faith it is impossible to please God, because..." Because? I never knew there was more to this Scripture. I read further, *"anyone who comes to him must believe that he exists and that he rewards those who earnestly seek him."* I'm on the Bible App, so I look to see what the King James Version says. *"But without faith it is impossible to please him: for he that cometh to God must believe that he is, and that he is a rewarder of them that diligently seek him."* Seeing the word "diligently" sent me straight to my Webster app. I learned the meaning of diligently as characterized by steady, earnest and energetic effort.

Through my heartbreak and heartache, I had been diligently seeking God, not even realizing it. Mainly because over the years, it was simply who I had become, a lover of His Word. Even with a broken heart, I knew that He sat with me in my hospital room, I knew that He walked with me to each and every medical test and He was there as the tears fell like the worst rainstorm ever. He was there as test results were read to comfort me in my confusion and distress. He stayed true to His Word that He would perfect those things that concerned me and that He would work all things together for my good. He was using me as a light and a testimony. What the enemy meant for evil, God meant it for my good.

Heart Spills

I was 48 and an active mommy; I was eating correctly, losing weight and keeping up with my biometrics. I was working hard at keeping my numbers low and I still had a stroke. This is my heart spill that I pray is helpful to others:

- Know the signs of a stroke.
- Keep your phone charged at all times.
- Set up medical information in your phone that can be reached even if your phone is locked.
- At the sign of an emergency, get help ASAP.
- Know yourself well enough to know when you are in a crisis.
- Follow all of your doctor's orders.
- Keep up with all of your doctor's appointments.
- Know your medication's name and dosage.
- Keep your squad informed about what's going on with you.
- When you don't feel well, say it.
- Practice self-care.
- Practice mindfulness.
- Meditate.
- Keep a journal; write when you feel your best.
- Complete therapy.

- Know what activities calm your spirit.
- This above all, to thine own self be true.
- Trust God.

Leadership Thoughts

At Xavier University, located in Cincinnati, Ohio, I received my master's degree in education and studied in their Education Administration and School Superintendent Program. All of my professors were amazing. One of the many concepts that stayed with me was the concept of servant leadership, where the main goal of the leader is to serve. Right now, I'm reading, *Leaders Eat Last* by Simon Sinek where he discusses the Circle of Safety. The Circle of Safety is a concept that says that a leader protects those in their circle and that in return those in the circle, employees would look out for their leader.

I've had time to reflect on my situation and here are some thoughts to ponder:

- If you know that a staff member is to be reassigned be courteous and let them know in a timely manner. Allow them time to seek a position at another location, if that is their desire.
- Don't wait until after an employee's work day has ended to send an email about a change in assignment.
- Provide at least 1-2 weeks for the employee to prepare for the move.

- When a teacher is reassigned to your building, reach out to them and have a conversation, with them, about their new schedule, class load and culture of the school building.
- When a teacher arrives on the first day have their needed items prepared for them: room keys, passwords, enabled badge, to enter and exit the building, work computer, phone etc. Offer a tour of the building and introduce them to the team that they will be working with.
- When an employee is returning from a traumatic event have some *compassion*. When they contact your office refrain from responding to them by saying, "I know about your situation." when they call and have questions.
- Enlist a *compassionate* group of employees to assist employees with information about FMLA, medial leave while they are dealing with life changing events.
- When Human Resources comes up with a leave plan, put the plan in writing for the employee and the company, honor that agreement going forward.

- We you code an employee "Leave/No Pay", have a servant leaders heart and notify them via email, US mail or phone call. Employees shouldn't be blindsided, especially if they are already dealing with serious health issues.
- If as a district you've decided to code an employee "Leave/No Pay" without their knowledge and later send them a bill for medical insurance, honestly sit back and ask if this was the right thing to do.
- Provide professional development on Servant Leadership. Encourage leaders to read *Leaders Eat Last* and learn more about the Circle of Safety.
- Finally, *In this era of practicing self-care don't be an organization that promotes wellness and then punishes employees when they become ill.*

My prayer is that my situation benefits another teacher, employee, who experiences a similar situation.

DILIGENTLY

But without faith it is impossible to please him: for he that cometh to God must believe that he is, and that he is a rewarder of them that diligently seek him.
Hebrews 11:6 (AKJV

Books I've Read Since November 2018

It's Not Supposed To Be This Way by Lysa TerKeurst

Success Through Stillness by Russell Simons

Becoming by Michelle Obama

Crushing by T.D. Jakes

Girl, Stop Apologizing by Rachel Hollis

Leaders Eat Last by Simon Sinek

What I'm Reading Next

Girl, Wash Your Face by Rachel Hollis

Don't Settle For Safe by Sarah Jakes-Roberts

Black Pain: It Just Looks Like We're Hurting by
Terrie M. Williams

My Tidal Playlist

- Lo Unico Que Quiero ~ Marcela Gandara, Marco Barrientos
- More, More, More ~ Joann Rosario
- The Call ~ Isabel Davis
- You Know My Name ~ Tasha Cobbs Leonard, Jimi Cravity
- King of Glory ~ Todd Dulaney (Featuring Shana Wilson-Williams)
- My One My All ~ Jesus Culture, Chris McClarney
- Do It Again ~ Elevation Collective, Travis Greene, Kierra Sheard
- I Hear You Say ~ Joann Rosario
- Pulling Me Through ~ Todd Dulaney
- Your Great Name ~ Todd Dulaney
- Made A Way ~ Travis Green
- How He Loves ~ David Crowder Band
- Excited ~ Jonathan McReynolds
- Lord You Are Good ~ Todd Galberth
- God Is Good ~ Jonathan McReynolds
-

Woman Evolve

I had a vision about this book. I was going to have *Diligently* completed and ready to take to Denver in July of 2019 and somehow, I was going to get it to Bishop TD Jakes, First Lady Serita Jakes, Pastor Sarah Jakes-Roberts and her sister Cora Jakes via their security team. Then, before I got on my flight home, I was going to make the links to purchase the book live. I thought, "I'm about to kill the game." Lol. But then things didn't work out how I saw them in my mind, the book wouldn't be ready. However, I was ready for my second year of attending the Woman Evolve Conference in Denver, Colorado hosted by Pastor Sarah Jakes-Roberts.

My highlight for Woman Evolve 2018 was during the Pajama Session on that Friday night. Imagine a megachurch sanctuary filled with women in pajamas, worshipping God. It was such a beautiful sight. The media team had prepared a video for us to watch after praise and worship that evening. It contained footage from the morning session with Pastor Sarah. I remember thinking, "They did that quick. How cool to recap the earlier session." As the video played on, I realized that it was a video depicting how the Woman Evolve Conference grew out of Woman Thou Art Loosed, the women's conference founded by Pastor TD Jakes. The emotions of the audience was elevating and then out of stage left came Bishop TD Jakes to the stage. I cried unto God thanking Him for this moment. Here on a stage in Denver stood a pastor who had preached and comforted me through many instances.

I heard God say to me, "Did you not think that I would make sure that you came here and not have to worry about anything?" I along with other women, that I didn't know grabbed hands as Bishop Jakes prayed over us about going to the next dimension in our lives. I arrived back at my hotel so full already from worship that I didn't know if I could handle the next day. The next day came and it was even more incredible than the previous day. Experiencing worship and watching Pastor Sarah so overcome with emotion realizing her vision come to pass took me off guard.

Traveling to Denver was different this year. I had no financial worries or concerns about this trip. My sons and I had just returned from AAU Nationals for 7th grade basketball in Greensboro, NC. The team my son plays on, Ohio Ballstars, placed 5th in the nation. I decided to have my younger son fly out with me to see the mountains and relax from basketball for a while.

For Woman Evolve 2019 I had signed up for the Inner Circle registration which allotted me an opportunity to meet Pastor Sarah at a Meet & Greet on Thursday night. On the way to church that evening my friend Robert, who had been my driver from my previous visit to Denver, told me to be careful because the elevation was different and with my health concerns, I needed to be cautious. Once I arrived at the church and saw the long line, I thought, "Well, I'll just wait." Within moments I felt extremely tired and left the line, went to the gift shop and then called an Uber to go back to my hotel. I was so tired that is was unbelievable. I contacted Robert to tell him how I felt, and he shared that it could possibly take a couple of days to adjust. I went back to my hotel room and prepared for Session One of the conference the next day.

Session One was a true worship experience. Immediately I wondered how I would manage handling my health concerns and all of my emotions. The Second Session was with Pastor Sarah and her dad, Bishop TD Jakes. I was sitting there listening to them and then I felt weird. It felt like I could hear my pulse on the right side of my body and the heartbeat seemed to get stronger and stronger. After the session I asked one of the conference volunteers if they had a nurse. She asked me if I was ok and I simply said, "Yes, I just need to ask someone a question." I'm not one for attention, so I was not going to cause alarm by telling her what I was really feeling.

Once I am in the medical area, I ask the nurse for my blood pressure to be taken because I wasn't feeling well. After the nurse took my pulse, she was nice and comforting to me, she asked me several things,

"Are you on medication? What medication are you on? Do you live here? Have you eaten today? How much water have you had?"

I was honestly so tired that I'm not sure if I answered everything. She did inform me that my blood pressure was high, that I needed to get out of the heat and that I needed to drink some water. She then gave me two cold bottles of water and informed me how I could leave the building while staying in the most shade. As I began to leave, she stopped me.

"I need you to drink a bottle of water before you leave." She stated.

"Ok.", I said as I twisted open the top.

"I hate to sound like your mother." She said. Her tone was very stern and to be honest I truly appreciated it because I didn't want to be in crisis so far from home.

That evening I went back to my room and went to straight to sleep. I woke up the next morning with a different mindset. I drank more water during the morning and attended the morning session and the first breakout session, that was facilitated by celebrity Stylist J Bolin, celebrity hair stylist Nakia Collins and Pastor Sarah, entitled Kingdom & the Culture. It was at this session that I met Dr. Anita Phillips, a therapist that I follow on Instagram. At this point I'm feeling better and returned back to my hotel room to prepare for the evening.

When I arrived on Saturday, to the Potter House-Denver, for the final session I was filled with expectancy. I came into the sanctuary ready to worship and unlike last year I had reserved my flight to depart for Monday. I knew that I would need the rest when I returned to the hotel. After Pastor Sarah spoke, we had a worship session with worship leaders from Texas, Dave and Nichole Binion. I felt as if they knew Jesus' direct phone number and email because once they sang the first note, the cries of women filled the atmosphere. It is bone chilling to think about it even now. Those cries of anguish and brokenness filled the room. There was a point during this session where I sat back in my chair and wept loudly, and I saw an image come before me. I He knelt on one knee before and I could see his white gown flowing. He began to speak to me.

"Arlinda, I knew you would come back to Denver. I've been waiting to tell you how proud I am of you for handling everything so graciously. You could have cussed people out, treated people badly and made negative posts on Facebook but you didn't. You handled it with grace. And Arlinda, I knew all of these things would happen to you. I was there with you at every step. During the tests and when the results were read, I was there. I needed to you to break so that I could fill you up again." Directly behind me there was a woman crying. I happened to have on a sleeveless V-necked dress. As she cried, I didn't move as I felt her tears drop on my back. God spoke again. "That's your mantel now. To carry the tears of other hurting women on your back. To show love, hope and light to every woman you encounter. Let go of what has happened to you and continue to move forward graciously."

I sat there and thought about leaving my classroom that I loved, going to a new school, having a stroke the first day at the new school and everything that happened afterwards that lead me to a mega-church sanctuary in Denver where we cried out about bruised heels still crushing serpents head. Through my tears there were so many women hurting and crying and I wondered, "God, what am I supposed to do in this moment?" There was a young lady in front of me on her knees crying and praying. I gently touched her, and I could feel her trembling as she cried. I vowed in that moment that I would comfort and pray over her until she was able to get on her feet. I'm so thankful for that moment with God and to be a blessing to another woman. Jesus you change everything.

Thank You

I thank each and every person that prayed for me and blessed my family as we endured a very rough time. I'm so thankful for amazing parents, James and Natalie McGlothin, who made sure their daughter was ok. To my brother James and his wife Inga, thank you for being a strong presence in my life. To my sister, Marlene, thank you for being my voice during a time when my voice and thoughts made no sense to me or anyone else. To my cousin Lora, your humor and knowledge of FMLA helped me so much. To my aunts, Aunt Christine, Aunt Arlinda, and Aunt Barbara, I've always looked up to each of you and your love for me during this time made me feel like a little girl again. To Stephanie and Ryan, you two knew early on that my faith was not where it should have been and you made sure, daily, that I knew that God had so much more for me, even if I couldn't see. Thank you, Calvin, for coming to check on me. To Scott, thank you for your love and support while I was in the hospital.

My nephew rocks! James thank you for the incredible meals that resembled what I ate while I was in the hospital, a bean burger, a sweet potato and unsweetened applesauce makes me so happy now. To my niece Jauna thank you for coming to hang out with your auntie. Thank you, Sicily, for bringing the crew and reducing me to tears. Thanks to Bob for coming over and keeping our home organized and our family sane.

My church family is the bomb.com. Thank you, Pastor Mike, Deacon Mike (My BFF), Lady Kisha Scruggs and Mama Scruggs for checking on me and praying for me. Enjoli thank for being there, talking me through and keeping me cute.

I was so blessed by constant words of encouragement from my friend Greg, I am so blessed by our friendship. Thanks to my work mom, Mrs. Irvin-Smith, for always checking on me and blessing our family with tokens of love. Thanks to Quay Bailey for several amazing years together in the classroom. Trust me, you were more than a Paraprofessional in our classroom. To the Del Prince family, I love you two so much and I am so thankful for you both being in my life and sharing my love of lavender gardens. To the members of the National Sorority of Phi Delta Kappa, Sigma Chapter thank you for loving me and praying for me. It felt so good to come back to a beautiful circle of love. I truly needed that. Thank you, Vince for incredible conversations and much needed laughter.

To every administrator that I have ever worked under, I appreciate all of the lessons that I've learned and the skills and knowledge that I've acquired. While I am no longer in a teaching position, I will continue to grow as a servant leader, and I will always advocate for children and their families. My experience both as an educator and as an educator in crisis has birthed a newness in me, to be a better person and a better leader.

My students have meant the world to me over the years. I pray that they all go forth and do amazing things. I pray that they've learned that even when things don't work out in certain situations that they still have to finish the task assigned to them and finish it strong. November 1 and November 2 were two of the hardest days of my life, when I had to leave a program and students that I so greatly loved and cared for. I appreciate all of the messages of love and appreciation from families who truly recognized that I wanted the absolute best for their children.

Jai, thank you for constantly reminding me that, "I am her" and teaching me to savor the cheesecake. Thank you, Jen for allowing Jai to hang out with us this summer. His humor has been a blessing to my healing

Finally, I want to thank God for my two amazing sons, Alex and Tyler. Tyler you had a rough time, in the beginning, and here lately you've become the "keeper of me", always recognizing when I have expended myself to the point of exhaustion. While you jokingly say, "Mom, you need to rest. You do so much for the family" You also make a point to play mindful music, bring me a blanket and encourage me to rest. Thank you!!!! Alex, I'm still trying to figure out how you were able to shut down the Emergency Room. What message did you send out? Lol. Thank you for taking care of me and your brother. When the moment came that I knew that I was in crisis, my first born was my first thought. I knew that you would find me and make sure that I was taken care of. I thank God for trusting me to be a mom to both of you and then trusting that you two would take care of me. We've had a lot of Mommy-Son-Son time and I'm so grateful for you both.

And we know that in all things God works for the good of those who love him, who have been called according to his purpose.
Romans 8:28 (NIV)

Brethren, I count not myself to have apprehended: but this one thing I do, forgetting those things which are behind, and reaching forth unto those things which are before,
I press toward the mark for the prize of the high calling of God in Christ Jesus.

Philippians 3:13-14 (KJV)

My brethren, count it all joy when you fall into various trials.
James 1:2 (NKJV)

Words From Arlinda

I'm a woman who always searches for the meaning of things. Many years ago, when I started reading Oprah's magazine, I read an article entitled, *What I Know For Sure*. Here's what I know for sure now. God knew all these things would happen and He equipped me for the response in eternity. About 13 years ago, I was surplused to a school that was closing. I was sent there during its last year in operation. To be surplused means that because of a reduction in student population or student's course selections, there was not an available teaching position for me in my subject area in my present school based on current numbers. How awesome of God to allow me to be sent to another school that sat on the same grounds, that I was sent to so many years ago. In obedience, I went to where I was reassigned, and had a stroke on my very first day. God knew that the journey with my employer had ended for me on that same ground that I was sent to close down another school years ago. Only this time, there was no return for me. I have amazing experiences and credentials, but now God wanted me totally to be faithful to Him and to seek Him diligently. He wanted me to fully realize Jeremiah 29:11 for my life and to see how my daily 6:33 a.m. prayers as I recited Matthew 6:33, The Prayer of Jabez and The Prayer of Serenity were working in my life.

Unbeknownst to me, God had been equipping me for years for such a time as this. My only response to God was, "Yes, Lord!" And to the world, "She's ready for everything that God has for her." It's been the longest seven months of my life; but I've lost a lot and gained so much more. I can honestly say, "And we know that all things work together for good, for those that love God and called according to his purpose" (Romans 8:28).

I thank everyone who has prayed for me and my family. I thank everyone for amazing tokens of thoughtfulness. I thank God who spared and cared for me. I am thankful that He is allowing me to testify to having and surviving a stroke. I am letting the world know that covered girls don't look like what they've been through. I'd encourage everyone to continue to diligently and earnestly seek God. His plans and gifts are perfect and what He has for you will completely blow your mind.

Because of Him, I am…

Arlinda

Connect with me on social media and on my websites.

www.lindarinsights.blogspot.com

www.lindarinsights.com

Twitter ~ @lindarinsights
Facebook ~ @lindarinsights
Instagram ~ @lindarinsightspublishing
Snapchat ~ @lindarinsights
Pinterest ~ @lindarinsights

To contact me for speaking engagements or to facilitate a writing or self-publishing workshop contact me at
lindarinsights@gmail.com

More Books By The Author

Ghetto Chick ©2009
#hespoilsme ©2016
Infused ©2019
My Daily Gratitude Journal @2019

www.ingramcontent.com/pod-product-compliance
Lightning Source LLC
Chambersburg PA
CBHW032009040426
42448CB00006B/556